PELVIC FLOOR

WORKOUT FOR

BEGINNERS

Revitalize Your Foundation, Unlocking
The Secrets To Pelvic Floor Wellness
Through Effective Exercises Strength,
Stability, Lifestyle Strategies And
Confidence

LAMBERT FETTERMAN

DISCLAIMER

The content in this book is offered only for general informative purposes. While every effort has been taken to guarantee the content's accuracy and completeness, the author and publisher accept no responsibility for any mistakes or omissions, or for the results of using the information given herein. The methods, recommendations, and directions in this book are not guaranteed to be appropriate for every person, and readers should exercise caution and seek professional counsel if required before undertaking any of the projects or techniques detailed in this book.

Table of Contents

CHAPTER 1 10

Understanding The Pelvic Floor 10

Explain The Anatomy......................11

   1. Muscles on the Surface: 11

   2. Muscles of Intermediate Strength: 11

   3. Muscles Deep: 12

Muscles And Functions 12

   1. Support:..................................13

   2. Sphincteric Regulation:..............13

   3. Sexual Purpose: 13

   4. Postural Control: 13

Common Issues And Conditions 14

   1. Incontinence: 14

   2. Prolapse of Pelvic Organs: 14

   3. Pelvic Ache:............................15

CHAPTER 2 16

Importance Of Pelvic Floor Health 16

Impact On Overall Well-Being...........16

Relation To Posture And Movement ...17

Influence On Daily Activities 18

CHAPTER 3 ....**20**

Getting Started With Pelvic Floor Exercises **20**

Preparing For Exercises **20**

Basic Breathing Techniques...............**21**

Initial Muscle Awareness **22**

   1. Isolation: **22**

   2. Visual Aids: **23**

   3. Biofeedback equipment: **23**

Gradual Advancement **23**

CHAPTER 4 ....**26**

Core Pelvic Floor Exercises...............**26**

Kegels And Their Variations **26**

   • Kegels:...................................**26**

   • Kegel variations: **27**

Bridge Exercises **27**

Pelvic Tilts And Rolls......................**28**

CHAPTER 5 ....**30**

Advanced Pelvic Floor Workouts **30**

Resistance Training **30**

Integration With Full-Body Exercises ..**31**

Balance And Stability Routines 32

Safely Moving Forward:.................32

Progress Reporting:.....................33

Seeking Professional Help:.............33

CHAPTER 6 36

Maintaining Pelvic Floor Health 36

Daily Practices...............................36

1. Pelvic Floor Exercises:...............36

Lifestyle Adjustments 38

2. Limit High-Impact Activities: 38

3. Clothes Options: 38

5. Regular Check-ups: 39

Follow-Up And Progress Tracking......39

1. Journaling: 39

2. Consultation: 39

3. Reassessments: 39

CHAPTER 7 40

Special Considerations For Different
Groups 40

Pregnant Women 40

Postpartum Recovery 41

Aging And Menopause 42

  Considerations in General: 43

CHAPTER 8 46

Common Mistakes And How To Avoid
Them 46

Overexertion And Underutilization.....46

  • Excessive Kegels:.......................46

  • Ignoring Rest Days:....................46

  • Ignoring Signs of Discomfort: 47

Proper Form And Technique 47

  • Proper Breathing: 47

  • Engaging the Correct Muscles: 47

  • Consistent Practice: 48

CHAPTER 9 50

Moving Forward: Long-Term Pelvic
Floor Health 50

Incorporating Exercises Into Daily
Routine..50

Seeking Professional Guidance 51

Staying Consistent For Optimal Results
....52

Conclusion 53

THE END 56

CHAPTER 1

Understanding The Pelvic Floor

The pelvic floor is an important aspect of human anatomy that is made up of a set of muscles that create a hammock-like structure at the base of the pelvis.

This sophisticated network of muscles, ligaments, and connective tissues supports numerous pelvic organs such as the bladder, uterus, and rectum. Anyone beginning a pelvic floor training adventure must first understand the anatomy and functioning of the pelvic floor.

Explain The Anatomy

The pelvic floor is made up of multiple layers of muscles, each having its purpose. Muscles are typically classified into three types:

1. Muscles on the Surface:

• These muscles constitute the outermost layer of the pelvic floor and are in charge of supporting the perineum.

• The bulbospongiosus and ischiocavernosus muscles are two examples.

2. Muscles of Intermediate Strength:

• These muscles, which are located between the superficial and deep layers of the pelvic floor, help to maintain the structural integrity of the pelvic floor.

• Intermediate muscles include the transverse perineal muscles.

3. Muscles Deep:

• The deepest layer contains muscles such as the levator ani, which supports the pelvic organs.

• The levator ani is split into three muscles: the pubococcygeus, puborectalis, and iliococcygeus.

Muscles And Functions

Understanding how the pelvic floor muscles work is critical for sustaining pelvic health. These muscles are essential for a variety of biological functions:

1. Support:

• The pelvic floor supports the pelvic organs and prevents them from descending or prolapsing.

2. Sphincteric Regulation:

• Pelvic floor muscles produce a supporting sphincteric system that aids in the regulation of urine and fecal continence.

3. Sexual Purpose:

• Pelvic floor muscles have a role in sexual function, assisting in arousal and orgasm.

4. Postural Control:

• These muscles help to maintain postural stability and support the spine.

Common Issues And Conditions

Pregnancy, childbirth, age, and obesity are among the variables that might affect pelvic floor health. The following are some of the most common difficulties and conditions related to pelvic floor dysfunction:

1. Incontinence:

• Stress and urge incontinence are frequent problems that occur when the pelvic floor fails to appropriately support the bladder.

2. Prolapse of Pelvic Organs:

• This happens when pelvic organs, such as the uterus or bladder, drop into the vaginal region as a result of weakening pelvic floor muscles.

3. Pelvic Ache:

Chronic pelvic pain may be caused by conditions such as pelvic floor tension and myofascial pain syndrome.

Understanding the pelvic floor's elements lays the groundwork for efficient pelvic floor workouts and exercises. It enables people to address particular difficulties while also working to improve the strength and functioning of these vital muscles.

CHAPTER 2

Importance Of Pelvic Floor Health

The pelvic floor, a bundle of muscles at the base of the pelvis, is critical in maintaining key biological activities. Recognizing its significance includes understanding its influence on general health, posture, mobility, and daily activities.

Impact On Overall Well-Being

The pelvic floor is essential for urine and bowel control, sexual function, and the support of the pelvic organs (bladder, uterus, and rectum). A firm and functioning pelvic floor is important for general physical wellness. In contrast, weaker or malfunctioning pelvic floor muscles may cause urine incontinence, pelvic organ prolapse, and sexual dysfunction.

Relation To Posture And Movement

Good posture and balanced movement are linked to a healthy pelvic floor. These muscles collaborate with the core muscles to provide stability and support to the spine, hips, and pelvis. When the pelvic floor is weak or unbalanced, it may impact posture and cause problems such as lower back discomfort or instability during movement.

Influence On Daily Activities

Walking, lifting, and even sitting comfortably depend on the strength and flexibility of the pelvic floor, which we frequently take for granted. Proper operation guarantees that these actions may be completed with ease, without pain or the danger of problems.

Exercises and workouts intended to develop and support these muscles are essential for maintaining a healthy pelvic floor. Kegel exercises, which target these muscles and improve their strength and flexibility, are common in introductory pelvic floor workouts.

Understanding the importance of pelvic floor health enables people to make proactive efforts to maintain and improve these muscles. Prioritizing pelvic floor health, whether via focused workouts, keeping excellent posture, or adopting healthy lifestyle behaviors, adds greatly to overall well-being.

CHAPTER 3

Getting Started With Pelvic Floor Exercises

The pelvic floor, a set of muscles located at the base of the pelvis, supports pelvic organs, controls bladder and bowel movements, and contributes to sexual health. Starting with exercises is a proactive step toward improved pelvic health for beginners aiming to build and maintain their pelvic floor.

Preparing For Exercises

It is important to see a healthcare expert before beginning any fitness plan, particularly if you have pre-existing health ailments or concerns.

When you're ready to start, select a comfortable, peaceful place where you won't be distracted. Consider wearing clothes that are loose and comfy that enable you to move freely.

Basic Breathing Techniques

Pelvic floor workouts need effective breathing strategies. Begin with deep inhaling to increase oxygen flow to your muscles. Sit or lay down comfortably, relax your shoulders, and take a long, belly-expanding breath through your nose. Exhale softly through your lips, letting your tummy gradually flex. Concentrate on relaxing and activating your diaphragm.

Initial Muscle Awareness

It is critical to understand how to activate and relax the pelvic floor muscles. To begin, identify these muscles. Consider halting the flow of pee in the middle; these are the muscles you'll be working on. It is important to stress, however, that this "stop and start" technique is just for initial awareness and should not be adopted into daily activities.

To improve muscular awareness, do the following:

1. **Isolation:** Sit comfortably and concentrate on the muscles in your pelvic region. Try not to tense your belly, buttocks, or thighs when contracting these muscles.

Hold the contraction for a few seconds before releasing it.

2. Visual Aids: For some novices, visual aids such as diagrams or instructional films may assist them in grasping the placement and function of these muscles.

3. Biofeedback equipment: If accessible, use biofeedback equipment to assist in feeling muscular spasms and relaxation. These devices can offer real-time data on muscle activation.

Gradual Advancement

Beginners should begin with easy exercises and work their way up. Excessive effort or doing too much too quickly may cause muscular strain.

Initially, prioritize consistency over intensity. As you gain confidence, you may progressively increase the time and intensity of your workouts.

Remember that while starting pelvic floor exercises, patience and consistent practice are essential. It is a process of increasing muscular awareness and progressively strengthening these muscles to improve overall pelvic health. Always get tailored advice from a healthcare practitioner to verify that these workouts are appropriate for your specific requirements and circumstances.

CHAPTER 4

Core Pelvic Floor Exercises

The pelvic floor is a set of muscles that support the pelvic organs, help with bladder and bowel control, and contribute to sexual function. Exercises that engage these muscles may improve their strength and endurance, benefiting overall pelvic health.

Kegels And Their Variations

• Kegels: These exercises include tightening and releasing the muscles of the pelvic floor. Begin by identifying the muscles, which you may accomplish by attempting to halt the flow of pee midway (note: this is not an exercise, but rather a method of locating the muscles).

Contract and hold for a few seconds after identifying them before releasing. This should be done multiple times. Check to see whether you're tensing your abdomen, thighs, or buttocks.

• Kegel variations: Kegels may be tweaked to suit various degrees of strength and endurance. Quick Kegels entail tightening and releasing the muscles quickly. Slow Kegels concentrate on holding the contraction for a lengthy period, eventually increasing to longer holds.

Bridge Exercises

• Lie on your back with your legs bent and your feet on the floor. Engage your pelvic floor muscles as you raise your hips off the ground, forming a straight line from your shoulders to your knees. Hold this stance for a few seconds before lowering your hips. This exercise works the pelvic floor as well as the glutes and core muscles.

Pelvic Tilts And Rolls

• Lying on your back with your legs bent, do pelvic tilts. Rock your pelvis back and forth gently, stimulating the pelvic floor muscles. This exercise helps to develop and stabilize these muscles.

• Pelvic rolls entail circling the pelvis, which aids in the release of tension and the improvement of pelvic flexibility.

Remember, it's critical to complete these exercises correctly and progressively increase the intensity as your muscles strengthen. Consistency is essential for improving pelvic floor strength and function. Before starting any new fitness regimen, always visit a healthcare practitioner, particularly if you have pre-existing pelvic health concerns.

CHAPTER 5

Advanced Pelvic Floor Workouts

A strong pelvic floor program includes more than just fundamental exercises; it also includes advanced workouts that target enhanced strength, stability, and integration with full-body motions.

Resistance Training

Resistance training is essential for improving pelvic floor strength. You may increase the intensity of your pelvic floor exercises by using resistance bands or other gym equipment. These exercises use resistance against the pelvic muscles to help them strengthen and tone.

Incorporating resistance helps to target particular regions while also increasing general muscular endurance.

Integration With Full-Body Exercises

Pelvic floor exercises are often combined with full-body routines in advanced pelvic floor workouts. When squats, lunges, deadlifts, and planks are coupled with targeted activation of the pelvic floor muscles, a full exercise is created. Including pelvic floor activation in these workouts improves core stability, balance, and general strength.

Balance And Stability Routines

Balance exercises, such as standing on one leg or utilizing stability balls, help to improve pelvic floor fitness dramatically. These routines target the core muscles while also activating the pelvic floor as a stabilizer. Balance improvement not only strengthens the pelvic floor but also reduces the chance of injury and improves total body coordination.

Safely Moving Forward:

Gradual development is essential in any fitness plan. To minimize strain or damage, it is important to go gradually from fundamental to more difficult activities.

The key to good advancement is consistency in practice and recognizing your body's limitations.

Progress Reporting:

Progress tracking is critical in an advanced pelvic floor training plan. It aids in testing muscular strength, endurance, and general fitness. Keeping track of your workouts, length, and any changes in muscle activation may give significant insights into your development.

Seeking Professional Help:

Consultation with a pelvic floor expert, physiotherapist, or skilled fitness trainer might be advantageous for individuals entering into advanced routines.

They can provide specific coaching, ensure perfect technique, and successfully and securely lead you through advanced workouts.

By including these advanced methods in your pelvic floor program, you will improve not just muscle strength and stability, but also general fitness and functional mobility.

The emphasis on advanced exercises in this chapter serves as a guide for people who are ready to step up their pelvic floor exercise program, guaranteeing a well-rounded approach to pelvic floor health and fitness.

CHAPTER 6

Maintaining Pelvic Floor Health

The pelvic floor is necessary for many body processes, and it is critical to maintain its health with regular routines and lifestyle changes.

Daily Practices

1. Pelvic Floor Exercises: Create a program that includes Kegels, bridges, and pelvic tilts. Begin with simple exercises and work your way up to more complex regimens.

2. Maintain excellent posture to relieve strain on the pelvic floor.

Maintain proper body alignment when standing, sitting, and walking.

3. Maintain a fiber-rich diet to avoid constipation, which may strain the pelvic floor muscles.

4. Hydration: Drink enough water to maintain general health and optimum muscular function.

5. Regular Bowel Movements: Maintain regular bowel movements to avoid tension on the pelvic floor muscles.

6. Maintain a healthy weight to relieve strain on the pelvic region.

7. Stress Management: Use relaxation methods to minimize pelvic floor strain caused by stress.

Lifestyle Adjustments

1. Lifting large things that may strain the pelvic floor should be avoided. Use suitable lifting methods if required.

2. **Limit High-Impact Activities:** High-impact workouts, such as leaping, may cause pelvic muscle tension. Incorporate low-impact workouts into your fitness routine.

3. **Clothes Options:** Wear comfortable, supportive clothes, particularly during activity, to give proper pelvic support.

4. Avoid straining when urinating or having bowel motions. While using the restroom, relax the pelvic floor muscles.

5. Regular Check-ups: Visiting a healthcare expert regularly may assist in monitoring pelvic floor health and treating any issues.

Follow-Up And Progress Tracking

1. Journaling: Keep a diary to chronicle your workouts, food, and any changes in symptoms or pain.

2. Consultation: Seek advice from a healthcare expert regularly, particularly if you are having chronic problems or pain.

3. Reassessments: Review your workouts regularly, changing intensity or routines as required.

CHAPTER 7

Special Considerations For Different Groups

When it comes to pelvic floor exercises, adapting routines to individual groups is critical for their efficacy and safety. Here's a closer look at some of these unique considerations:

Pregnant Women

The pelvic floor is affected by considerable changes in a woman's body during pregnancy. Exercises should concentrate on gradual strengthening and maintaining pelvic floor function throughout this period to assist the expanding uterus and prepare for delivery.

, pelvic tilts, and adapted prenatal yoga may help with strengthening and relaxation. However, it is critical to seek personalized advice from a healthcare provider because certain exercises may not be appropriate at all stages of pregnancy.

Postpartum Recovery

The pelvic floor is strained and perhaps traumatized after delivery. Gradual re-strengthening exercises, such as gentle Kegels and pelvic floor relaxation techniques, are frequently prescribed to help with recovery. This aids in the restoration of muscle tone, the prevention of incontinence issues, and the overall recovery. Postpartum physical therapy can provide customized exercises to address specific needs during this time.

Aging And Menopause

Hormonal changes associated with aging and menopause can have an impact on pelvic floor health, resulting in issues such as weakened muscles and increased susceptibility to prolapse or incontinence. Exercises that focus on strengthening and maintaining elasticity become critical. Pelvic floor awareness, core stability, and overall fitness routines all contribute to pelvic floor health as part of an active lifestyle.

Considerations in General:

Regardless of the group, it is critical to proceed with caution and under professional supervision when performing pelvic floor exercises, especially if there are pre-existing health conditions or concerns. Universal principles include emphasizing proper form, avoiding excessive strain, and allowing adequate recovery time between exercises. Furthermore, understanding one's own body and its limits is critical for avoiding overexertion or injury.

Consultations with healthcare professionals or specialists, such as physiotherapists or gynecologists, can provide personalized guidance, ensuring exercises are appropriate for individual needs and health conditions.

Furthermore, modifying exercises based on comfort levels and gradual progression helps to prevent strain or injury, ensuring a sustainable and beneficial pelvic floor health routine throughout different life stages.

CHAPTER 8

Common Mistakes And How To Avoid Them

In pelvic floor exercises, proper form and technique are critical. Here's a comprehensive guide to avoiding common blunders and mastering techniques:

Overexertion And Underutilization

• **Excessive Kegels:** Excessive Kegel exercises can strain the pelvic floor muscles. Prioritize quality over quantity, and allow for relaxation between contractions.

• **Ignoring Rest Days:** Muscles require time to recover. Avoid doing intense workouts on consecutive days. Alter your workout days with rest or light exercise days.

• **Ignoring Signs of Discomfort:** Pain or discomfort during exercise may indicate poor form or overstrain. Stop immediately if you feel any discomfort.

Proper Form And Technique

• **Proper Breathing:** Improper breathing can interfere with pelvic floor engagement. Avoid holding your breath during exercises by breathing naturally.

• **Engaging the Correct Muscles:** Make sure you're targeting the pelvic floor muscles rather than the abdominal or thigh muscles. Concentrate on isolating and contracting these muscles.

- **Consistent Practice:** Regular, consistent workouts are more effective than intense sessions on occasion. Create and stick to a routine.

CHAPTER 9

Moving Forward: Long-Term Pelvic Floor Health

Incorporating Exercises Into Daily Routine

The foundation of pelvic floor health is daily routines. By incorporating specific exercises into your daily routine, you can ensure consistency and gradual progress. Begin by allocating specific time each day for these exercises. Incorporate them into your morning or evening routines to make them a habitual part of your day. The importance of consistency in strengthening and maintaining pelvic floor muscles cannot be overstated.

Seeking Professional Guidance

While beginner exercises are accessible, seeking professional guidance offers significant benefits. Consultation with a pelvic floor physiotherapist or specialist helps personalize exercises based on your individual needs. These professionals can assess your muscle strength and offer tailored exercises that address specific weaknesses or imbalances. They also provide valuable insights into posture corrections and lifestyle adjustments that contribute to pelvic floor health.

Staying Consistent For Optimal Results

Consistency is fundamental in achieving and maintaining pelvic floor health. Even after mastering the beginner exercises, it's crucial to sustain these practices for long-term benefits. Regularity ensures that your pelvic floor muscles remain strong and functional. Maintain consistency not only in the exercises but also in lifestyle choices that support pelvic floor health, like maintaining proper hydration, avoiding excessive straining during bowel movements, and incorporating healthy habits.

Conclusion

Understanding the importance of pelvic floor exercises is crucial for beginners. These exercises promote pelvic floor health and overall well-being. Throughout this workout journey, beginners become acquainted with the anatomical structure and function of the pelvic floor muscles. The workouts start with basic exercises like Kegels, gradually advancing to more complex routines for increased strength and flexibility.

It's essential to avoid common mistakes that could hinder progress, such as overexertion or improper form. By maintaining a consistent routine, individuals can observe improvements in their pelvic floor health, leading to enhanced posture, and stability, and reduced risks of pelvic floor-related issues.

Long-term maintenance is vital. By integrating exercises into their daily routines, individuals can sustain the health benefits achieved through consistent workouts. Seeking guidance from healthcare professionals or specialists ensures proper form and technique, reducing the risk of injury.

In conclusion, the journey to pelvic floor health is ongoing. Beginners learn that regular exercises, proper technique, and seeking professional advice contribute to maintaining optimal pelvic floor health for the long term. The commitment to a consistent routine ensures the continued well-being of the pelvic floor muscles, enhancing overall health and functionality.

THE END